"Kim is an accomplished personal trainer who skillfully uses her sense of humor to motivate people to exercise. That humor is evident in Gym Etiquette 101, yet when reading between the lines, we are reminded that exercise is holistic. Strengthen and tone the body and relax the mind....leave that social media behind!"
> ~Rosalind Becker, PA-C,
> Physician Assistant Studies director and university professor

"The definitive guide to gym etiquette. I thought I knew everything I needed to know about this subject until now. It made me laugh out loud and inspired me at the same time. Worth the read and definitely on my next book list to read again."
> ~Steve Hicks, songwriter, gym advocate,
> Dockwood Music owner and instructor

Kim Becknell Williams

Gym Etiquette 101

Written by Kim Becknell Williams, CPT
Illustrated by Sloane Williams

Kim Becknell Williams

I dedicate Gym Etiquette 101 to my family for their endless support during the five years it took to write this book. It really does take a village or at least a village of family.

The illustrations in this book were drawn by my niece, Sloane Williams. Many thanks to her for sharing her artistic talents and quick wit in creating the illustrations, as well as the cover. Find her artwork at: Asloanewilliams.wix.com/a-little-to-the-left.

Disclaimer: The author has made every effort to ensure that the information contained in this book is complete and accurate at the time of its publication. However, neither the author nor the publisher is rendering any time of professional advice, medical advice or health care services to the individual reader. You should consult with your personal physician or health care professional before beginning, resuming or modifying any exercise program. All matters regarding your health or any exercise program require medical supervision. Neither the author nor the publisher shall be liable for any loss, injury or damage allegedly arising from any information, opinions or suggestions contained in this book. Neither the author nor the publisher has any continuing obligation to update any information contained in this book as new discoveries, research or information becomes available. The author's references to various products are for information purposes only and are not intended as an endorsement of those products by the author or the publisher.

Table of Contents

"When you become a believer in yourself you are on the road that leads to where you want to go." ~ Norman Vincent Peale[1]

Introduction: The reason I wrote this book

Years ago, I had to quit playing tennis. I had been on five tennis teams, but work demands took over and I had to throw in the tennis towel. So, I turned to the gym with its flexible hours and started a new exercise routine. It was all new to me and I didn't know what to expect, but I had to try. I wanted to stay in shape.

I pushed my cute tennis clothes to the back of the closet and shopped for appropriate gym clothes. It was a whole new world, but I still wanted to make sure that I felt good about what I wore. Tennis teams (at least the ones I was on) take great effort in choosing uniforms. I wanted to find cute gym attire since my tennis clothes had been retired.

Next, I wanted to make sure I developed a habit of exercising. I packed my exercise clothes, water bottle and shoes the night before work. I carried my gym bag into my office and set it under my desk. Once the work day ended, the workout day began. By changing at work and driving directly to the gym, I had no distractions to sidetrack me.

Eventually, I learned how to use the equipment by watching others and asking for help. I tried some classes, including Zumba, strength training and yoga. I found what I enjoyed the most. There were no fancy gym lunches

---

[1] The Power of Positive Thinking, pg. 18, Norman Vincent Peale

like after tennis matches, but I did start to get to know some fellow gym members.

Then, I injured my shoulder using an ab board on a wooden floor. I tore it up really bad, had surgery, seven months of physical therapy and a long recovery. When the surgeon told me I would have an 18-month recovery, it sounded like an eternity. I dug my heels in and gained determination for the long haul.

Three days after the surgery, I was at the gym with my arm in a sling. My husband stood by me while I rode the stationary bike to make sure I didn't fall off, still groggy from the anesthesia. I didn't bike for long, but I did it. It was the affirmation I needed to know...I could keep at it even in a sling.

As the weeks and months went by, I had to be creative with my workout to dodge my shoulder issues. In the process, I tried new equipment, varied my exercises and kept at it religiously.

The result? I was in better shape than I was when I played on five tennis teams. And, I became a certified personal fitness trainer in honor of my fiftieth birthday. I feel the reasons why I was in better shape, were:

- I varied the types of exercises that I did, so I used different muscles. This threw my body off of schedule, so it worked harder to burn calories. And it kept me from getting bored.
- Adding weights improved my fitness level.
- I worked every muscle in my body.
- With the flexible hours, I never had a reason not to go: 5 a.m. before work or 5 p.m. after work. Sometimes, I worked in two-a-days.
- I didn't have to wait to find a teammate to do it. I could go to the gym all by myself.
- On weekends, I'd use the extra time to lengthen my workouts.
- I had fun, so I wanted to do it more.

In many ways, joining and working out at the gym saved my sanity. Giving up tennis and damaging my shoulder could have ended my exercise career. But, it didn't.

At first I was unsure of how the gym would benefit me. Now, the gym is where I go to forget the rest of the world. And it's where I go to take care of me mentally and physically.

I have spent many, many hours at the gym. My observations over the years, combined with conversations I've had with other gym rats,[2] provide the background material for Gym Etiquette 101. So, in effect, I've been doing research all along. I have found lots of humor in my time at the gym too, so I've included some of that. I hope you enjoy reading the book as much as I enjoyed writing it.

See you at the gym,
Kim Becknell Williams

---

[2] www.urbandictionary.com defines a gym rat as "One who spends entirely too much time partaking in muscle building, strength training, cardiovascular or aerobic activity. Specifically, one who does so at a health club or gym."

"Fitness – if it came in a bottle, everybody would have a great body."
~ Cher [3]

The starting line

As a former sprinter in school, I still think in running terms. So, we begin at the starting line...

The starter shouts "on your mark." Your feet are in the blocks with your hands resting on the track for support. Set! You raise your rump up to prepare to come out of the blocks with finesse and speed. The starter's gun sounds and you're off.

You are in the race, this human race. Might as well make it a good one. Welcome to Gym Etiquette 101 – a simple class inside this book. There is no test at the end and no one is keeping score, except for you. Within the pages, 10 tips help you to learn about working out in a gym.

A gym is much like an adult playground, so you'll want to make sure you can get along with others in the proverbial sandbox.

Just like going out to dinner or standing in line to pay for groceries, there are boundaries and manners at the gym. You don't spit your gum out on the table at dinner; and you don't break in line to pay for groceries. Well, hopefully you don't. If you do, there are some other books you might need to be reading.

This book is your own personal guide to learn the basics of what to expect when you walk through the doors of a typical gym. Journals and charts are

---

[3] www.quotationpage.com/collections, from Laura Moncur's Motivational Quotations

provided for you to keep a record of your thoughts and activities along the way.

Many people are intimidated by a gym and either never give it a try or give up too soon. Every January, I watch as a huge influx of people who have created New Year's Resolutions invade the gym. I watch every February as these same people drop out.

With the helpful tips in this book, I hope you won't be one that drops out a month into your journey. Ideally, you'll find a perfect fit in the gym for a lifetime supporting healthy habits.

And if you do drop out, it doesn't have to be permanent. My intention is for this book to remind you that you can always start over with a whole new beginning.

There is always room for you at the starting line.

If you already exercise in a gym, you'll recognize some characteristics and might learn a thing or two. And if you do use a gym regularly, you have probably discovered the value.

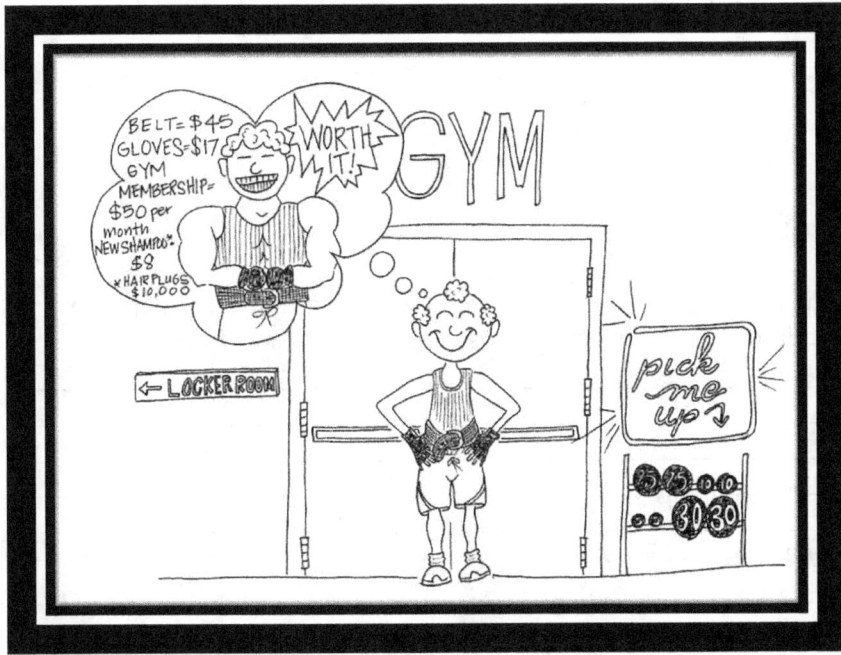

According to gym rats, a gym provides many benefits:
- Even if the weather is bad, you can exercise.
- Working out with others can be energizing and very motivating.
- A gym will keep you up to date on new ways to exercise.
- A gym provides the opportunity for variety in your exercise routine.
- Instructors and trainers can show proper techniques to prevent injury.
- You can wear new workout clothes. ☺
- By going away from home to exercise, you can de-stress from the daily routine.
- Competition with others can encourage you. Competition with yourself can too.
- A gym provides a sense of community with people who have a common interest.
- It refocuses the day/night and puts it in a healthy frame of mind.
- Working out at a gym can help with maintaining a healthy weight.

Now, fill in five of your own reasons or choose what you feel are the most important from the list above. Writing it down will register it with your brain.

1.
2.
3.
4.
5.

G – Get
Y – Your
M – Motivation

What is the reason you exercise? Do you want to get more fit? Improve a health condition? Train for a race? Lose weight? Just have fun?

_____

_____

_____

_____

_____

How will you stay motivated?

_____

_____

Gym Etiquette 101

Music keeps me motivated when I'm exercising. I switch the songs around on my iPod to be suited to each particular exercise. If I want to hold in plank for two minutes, I find a song that lasts that length of time.

My personal favorites (which are always changing and evolving) to help me step it up include:

- "Push It" by Salt-n-Pepa
- "Moneytalks" by AC/DC
- "Uptown Funk" by Bruno Mars and Mark Ronson
- "Der Kommissar" by After the Fire
- "U Can't Touch This" by MC Hammer
- "Bad Medicine" by Bon Jovi
- "Come With Me Now" by KONGOS

And when I need to slow it down for lifting weights or stretching, I might tune into:

- "The Hanging Tree" by James Newton Howard
- "Cool Kids" by Echosmith
- "Habits" by Tove Lo
- "Drink In My Hand" by Eric Church
- "FourFiveSeconds" by Rihanna, Kanye West and Paul McCartney
- "Beer On The Table" by Josh Thompson
- "Take Me To The River" by Talking Heads

Find your own playlist to get your groove on.

Some people post pictures of themselves at the size or fitness level they once were on their refrigerators. This gives them a visual image of what they can strive for again. Guess they could carry that picture with them in a gym bag for reference and continued motivation.

Whatever your motivation is, turn your exercise routine into a fun workout. If it's fun, you're most likely to stick with it. According to statisticbrain.com, the Centers for Disease Control and Prevention[4]:

---

[4] Statisticbrain.com, Research date: July 8, 2014, Source: Centers for Disease Control

- 60% of Americans don't get the recommended 30 minutes of exercise 5 days a week
- 25% of adults aren't exercising at all

But,

- 45,300,000 Americans have gym memberships
- 29,750 health clubs exist in the U.S.

One might conclude that people join gyms, but don't use them adequately. What's up with that? Is it good break room discussion to say you're a member at a gym? Does it impress people? Does it make the person feel like they are making an effort toward good health? Or do they join a gym and enter the doors only to find out they don't know what to do?

Look around you at the gym and you'll see people of all ages and sizes who are working on their fitness level. Young, old, fit, not quite fit, skinny, overweight, physically disabled – they're all there and they're all trying to improve. Hopefully they enjoy the workout while working on their fitness level. It shouldn't be drudgery to get out and get fit. And it is possible to smile while you exercise. So, smile and pick up that dumbbell.

"Those who think they have not time for bodily exercise will sooner or later have to find time for illness." ~ Edward Stanley[5]

#gymfails

Using social media, I recently polled gym rats and found the top 15 pet peeves (marked as #gymfails in this book):

1. Not wiping down equipment (the biggest complaint by a landslide)
2. Lifting and caveman-type grunting
3. Not re-racking weights
4. Talking on the phone while using equipment
5. Watching other people exercise
6. Leaving wet towels in the locker room/sauna
7. Walking into classes late
8. People talking to you while you're exercising
9. Provocative dressing
10. Hogging equipment
11. The arrogant walk, cocky strutting
12. People who stink
13. Those trying to find a "hook up"
14. Germs brought into the gym
15. Slamming weights down to get noticed

I saw a woman the other day that hit the trifecta in #gymfails. She was on her phone posing in front of the mirror while blocking the bosu balls (looks like half of a balance ball with a sturdy base).

---

[5] 5 www.goodreads.com/quotes/173133

In another poll, I created an online survey conducted through Survey Monkey® (Jan. – Feb. 2015), to collect information about the general public's thoughts and intimidations about gyms and exercise in general.

The respondents were 74% female and 26% male all over the age of 18. Most of them, 95%, had visited a gym; 5% had never walked in the doors of one. They answered the questions anonymously. The results were part of the research done for this book. The following graphs and charts show a summary of the results.

How important is exercise to you?

Very important	39%
Extremely important	31%
Moderately important	22%
Slightly important	6%
Not at all important	2%

All but 2%, that's 98%, see some importance in exercise. How would you rate yourself? Circle your answer below.

- Extremely important

- Very important

- Moderately important

- Slightly important

- Not at all important

How often do you exercise?

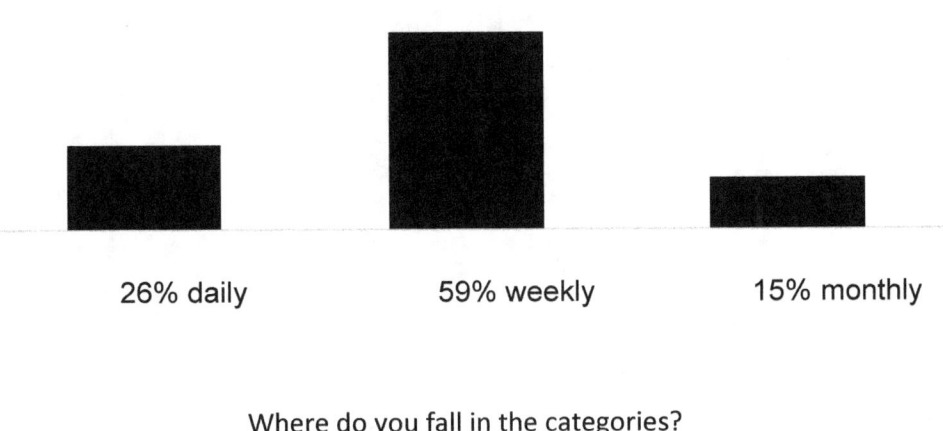

26% daily   59% weekly   15% monthly

Where do you fall in the categories?

_____

If you have been to a gym or thought about going to one, what appeals most to you?

65% - The variety of equipment and classes appeals to me most.

24% - Being around other people motivates me to exercise.

18% - Even in bad weather, I can exercise in a gym.

10% - Other: attitude, environment, personal training, swimming pool, structure, safety

Fun Fact: Variety is the spice of the gym life.

What intimidates you about working out in a gym?

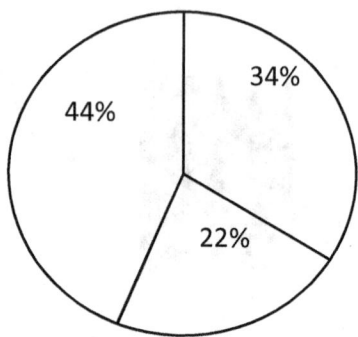

44% nothing intimidates me

34% not knowing how to use the equipment or
what is involved with classes

22% being around fit people and feeling bad about myself

More than half, 56%, are intimidated by something at a gym.

Does something intimidate you at the gym? If so, what?

_____

_____

_____

_____

What quality is most important at a gym?

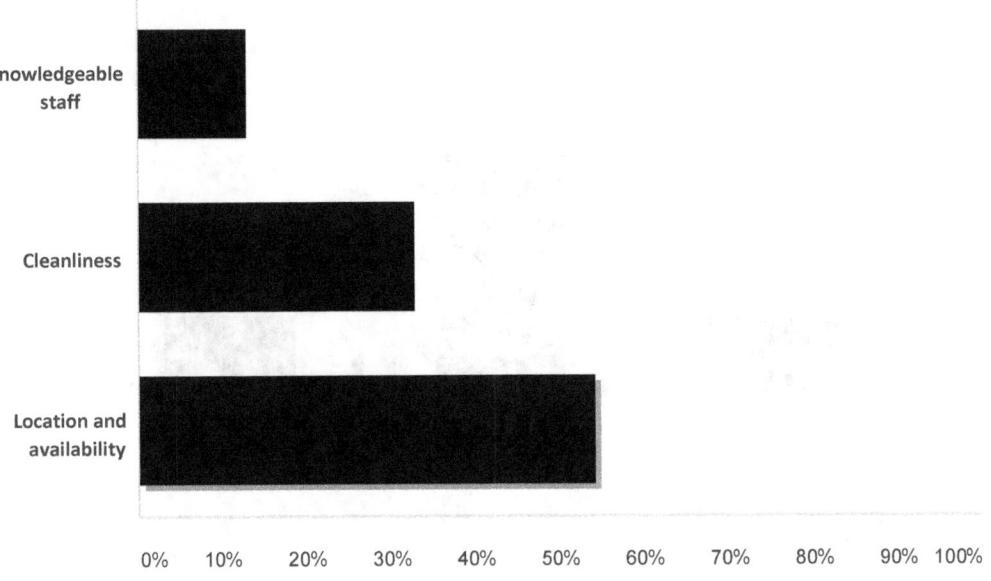

More than half, 54%, feel location and availability are most important.

What's most important to you?

- Knowledgeable staff
- Cleanliness
- Location and availability
- Other _____

I consider my fitness level to be

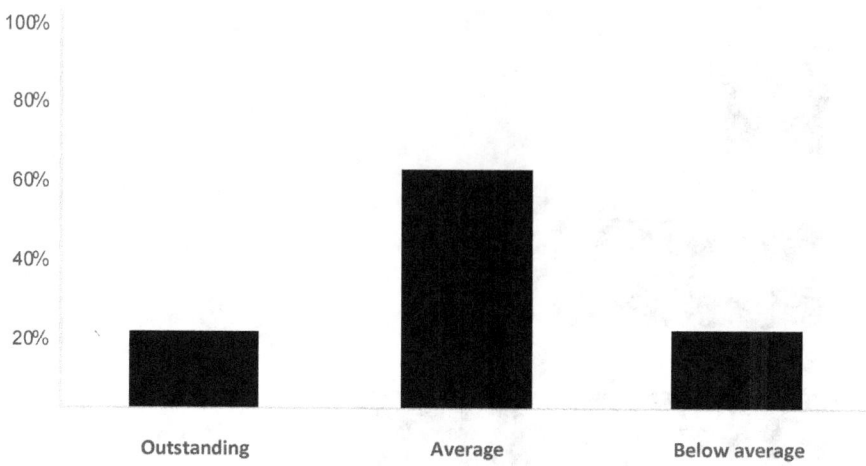

Is average good enough?

Where does your fitness level rank?

- Outstanding

- Average

- Below average

I would like to improve my fitness level.

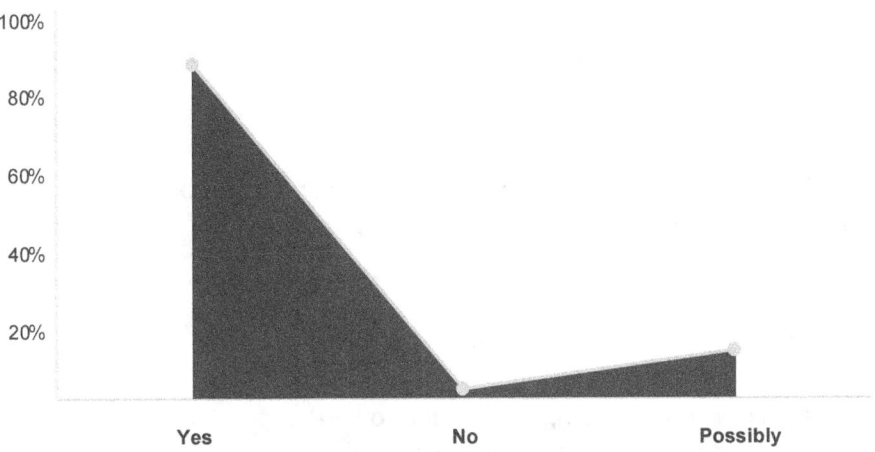

Everyone had some level of interest in improving their fitness level. Even those who exercise daily and consider their fitness level to be outstanding, want to improve their fitness level.

The journey in the gym never really stops.

Pack your mental suitcase for the trip. It will be a wild ride. But before you start the ignition, we move into our gym tips to throw intimidation out the window.

"Motivation is when you get hold of an idea and don't let go of it until you make it a reality." ~ Dr. Wayne Dyer[6]

Tip 1

Choose the right gym

Joining a gym is a step in the right direction toward improving fitness. Before you join, choosing the right one is crucial.

This may seem like a no brainer, but you should arm yourself with information about what you want and be clear about it BEFORE sitting down to talk with a gym representative. The gym rep may or may not have your best interest at heart, oftentimes, being very persuasive in convincing people to join. Their paycheck could depend on it.

I have been in a work environment where gym reps came in to give group employee discounts on gym memberships. The peer pressure was intense and the rep kept pushing. Most of the employees joined and all of them dropped their memberships within a few months.

Shopping for a gym is similar to buying a car or a house. Doing your homework ahead of time can be very helpful. You're making an investment in your health, so it is vital.

Be aware of special programs that might be offered, like medical discounts (if appropriate). Usually these require a doctor's signature, but can provide guidance in nutrition and exercise in addition to a reduced rate. Another program offered nationally at various gyms is the Silver Sneakers program.

---

[6] Family Circle, *Seven Secrets of a Joyful Life*, June 2005

Gym Etiquette 101

This is only for people over the age of 65 and only with specific insurance carriers, but is offered at a minimal cost. Instructors are specifically trained to work with this age group. Check the Silver Sneakers website to see eligibility guidelines.

If you've never been to a gym before, you might want to visit as many gyms (with memberships within your monetary budget) as you can to get a good perspective. Most gyms offer one or more free visits to potential members.

Try out their classes. Spend time in the general exercise areas. If you swim, try the pool.

There are big and subtle differences in gyms.

Some older gyms still have separate exercise rooms for men and women...yep, really.

Hours can vary; a few gyms stay open 24/7. Who wants to do box jumps at 3 a.m.? Must be someone out there who exercises in the wee hours of the morning.

On the contrary, some gyms have very limited hours.

Talk to people who exercise at the gyms and get their opinions on their experience. Most importantly, choose a gym where you feel comfortable. It has to "feel" right to keep you coming back.

Follow the checklist provided here based on YOUR needs and you'll be ready to make your own decision. Three are provided here, so you can compare at the end of your gym tour. More copies of the checklist are included at the end of the book.

Look at the categories in the far left column and cross out any subject that doesn't matter to you. For the remaining subjects, rate them on a scale of 1 – 4 using the following criteria. Write the number in the second column.

1 = poor
2 = fair
3 = good
4 = excellent

The third column provides space for your comments. Total the score and write it beside the gym name for future reference to determine the right gym for you.

Gym name _____Score_____

Category	Rating	Comments
Location		
Hours		
Variety of programs, classes		
Child care		
Atmosphere		
Helpful staff, instructors		
My comfort level while there		

Gym name _____Score_____

Category	Rating	Comments
Location		
Hours		
Variety of programs, classes		
Child care		
Atmosphere		
Helpful staff, instructors		
My comfort level while there		

Gym Etiquette 101

Remember, before signing on the dotted line for any gym membership, to make sure you can cancel at any time without penalty. Read the fine print.

Gym name _____Score_____

Category	Rating	Comments
Location		
Hours		
Variety of programs, classes		
Child care		
Atmosphere		
Helpful staff, instructors		
My comfort level while there		

Assuming you've made your decision on which gym to join, now it's time to get to know the ins and outs at your new exercise facility.

"Starting a new way is never easy so…keep starting until the start sticks."
~Tim Fargo[7]

Tip 2

Navigate your gym

There is no reason to drive around the parking lot looking for the closest parking space at the gym. The whole point in an exercise program is…drumroll please…to exercise. Park your vehicle in the back of the lot and walk your way into the gym. Each step counts! If it's raining, you'll cool off on your way back to your car.

One sunny day, I witnessed two women arguing over a parking space in the gym parking lot. There was plenty of parking available, just not close to the entrance. They had no children with them and didn't appear to be injured at all. I guess they forgot the purpose in going to a gym…exercise!

Once you've chosen the right gym, parked your car and walked in the door, it's time to familiarize yourself with the entire gym. Start with the basics: locate the bathrooms, water fountain, coffee pots, locker rooms and help desk. Where's the pool? Are lanes designated for certain swimmers?

- Find out where the antibacterial spray/towels are located. That's the #1gymfail in our pet peeve list.
- You don't want to be on a machine with a sudden urge to pee and not know where the bathrooms are located.
- Some water fountains will have an extension feature on them allowing easier water bottle refill.

---

[7] www.goodreads.com/quotes/1019155

- Make sure there are combination or key locks on the lockers, if you choose to use them. Theft exists everywhere, locker rooms included.
- Many locker rooms provide overhead or portable hair dryers, hygiene supplies, as well as bathing suit drying machines.
- If you need to bandage a blister or a cut, have a question or feel light-headed, you'll need to know where to get help.

Next, survey the workout areas and rules. Sometimes the popular equipment will have sign-up sheets/white boards with time limitations. You don't want to jump in line, especially with a linebacker-looking dude in front of you.

Find out where the free weights are so you can incorporate them as needed. Using them can be a time-filler while waiting for a class to begin or while waiting to use equipment. There's no point in just standing around. Make every minute count. You might want to check the weight on each dumbbell to make sure you reach for what you want; there's a big difference in 8 – 25 – 60, etc. Depending on the way they are made, it can be difficult to determine weight just by looking at it. The number of pounds will be imprinted usually on the end of the dumbbell. Kettlebells, similar to a dumbbell with a handle on it, will have their weight on them also.

Be sure to return the weights. Not re-racking weights is a no-no. #gymfail3 Know where the stretching areas are, as well as mats and stretching yoga-type bands. Balance balls are great to incorporate in your routine. Doing crunches on one is much more challenging than doing them on the floor. Like re-racking weights, be sure to return mats and exercise toys to their storage locations.

If you choose to take classes, find out where they are taught and if you need to bring anything: yoga mat, free weights, etc. Oftentimes the popular classes require signing up ahead of time and/or bringing a ticket, which prevents overcrowding. Check with the gym workers to find out before you decide to take a class.

When you take a new class, let the instructor know before the class begins that it's your first time. The instructor can help guide you. Workshops or introductory classes may also be offered for beginners. Be on time for class, which will ensure a good spot on the floor. Being late is taboo and many lock the door once class has started. #gymfail7

Try new classes until you find what you like. Amy Prasol, a certified Zumba instructor since 2007, teaches Zumba and other types of classes, including kickboxing, in the Boston, Massachusetts area. "I always tell people when it's the first class they're taking of mine and they're trying to get involved in fitness that they need to keep trying everything," Prasol said. "Soon they will find something they love and then it won't seem like work."

Take a friend along, which can be a huge support system. You can keep each other accountable.

Here's a brief description, from my point of view, of classes I have tried or observed. New classes are popping up all the time, so do your research ahead of time if there's something you haven't heard of before. Instructors may make variations to their individual class instruction.

- Zumba classes involve dance rhythms typically with Latin music. The dance moves can quickly change, so lighten up on yourself if it takes a while to learn the moves or if you fall. I was in a class once where a woman fell flat on her back; and she was in the front row. Once I knew she was okay, I couldn't stop thinking about it and got the giggles!
- Yoga, which is said to have originated in India, incorporates "postures" to strengthen and stretch. There are many types and levels of yoga, so research your class ahead of time. Please note: if you decide to take a hot yoga class, do not eat much beforehand. People have vomited during the class from eating too much before taking hot yoga. Yuck!
- Pilates incorporates equipment and yoga-type moves.
- Strength conditioning uses various weights during the workout. Be sure to follow the instructor for proper form. I always find new muscles I didn't know I had after taking these classes.
- Spin classes, aka cycling, use stationery bikes for a solid cardio and leg workout. Some classes provide virtual scenery to make it seem like you're biking outdoors in fabulous places like the Grand Canyon or the Swiss Alps. I have seen puddles of sweat on the floor, so if you're one who sweats a lot, carry your towel with you.

- Kickboxing involves lots of punching and kicking.
- Water aerobics is said to be easy on the joints and provides a safe exercise that benefits all parts of your body. Water-type weights and equipment are oftentimes used to provide resistance.
- Suspension training uses hanging or pulling straps to perform exercises.
- Plyometric exercise involves lots of jumping, lunges and squats with changes in direction during the exercises for an intense workout.
- Boot camp is usually a tough, sweaty class that incorporates cardio and strength training for a vigorous workout. Classes may be held outdoors or indoors or a combination of both.
- Barre classes incorporate a ballet barre or ballet-type exercises for a serious workout.

The popularity of exercise classes seems to move in waves. Whatever the rage is right now will probably not be the same in a few months. So, the size of classes can vary. Don't be discouraged by a crowd; next week it could change. And if it's a really small class, you'll get extra attention. Have you tried exercise classes before? Which ones did you like and why?

_____
_____
_____
_____

Were there classes that you didn't like and why not?

_____
_____
_____

_____

Is there an indoor or an outdoor track at your gym? If so, find out the distance around the track. Walking and/or running can always be incorporated into your routine. Some indoor tracks have rules for which direction to walk/run in, as well as which lanes are designated for walkers/runners. Check for any rules before you begin.

Do you like to walk or run? Y/N? Inside/Outside?

Is there a gymnasium to shoot hoops? Are there organized basketball games or pick-up games? Do you need to check-out a basketball from the front desk?

Kim Becknell Williams

Are tennis courts or racquetball courts available? Where are the sign-ups for court reservations?

Is there a sauna/hot tub? Does the gym provide towels?

Learning your way around can be like a pirate following a treasure map. Instead of walking the plank, you'll be doing the plank.

Your booty will thank you!

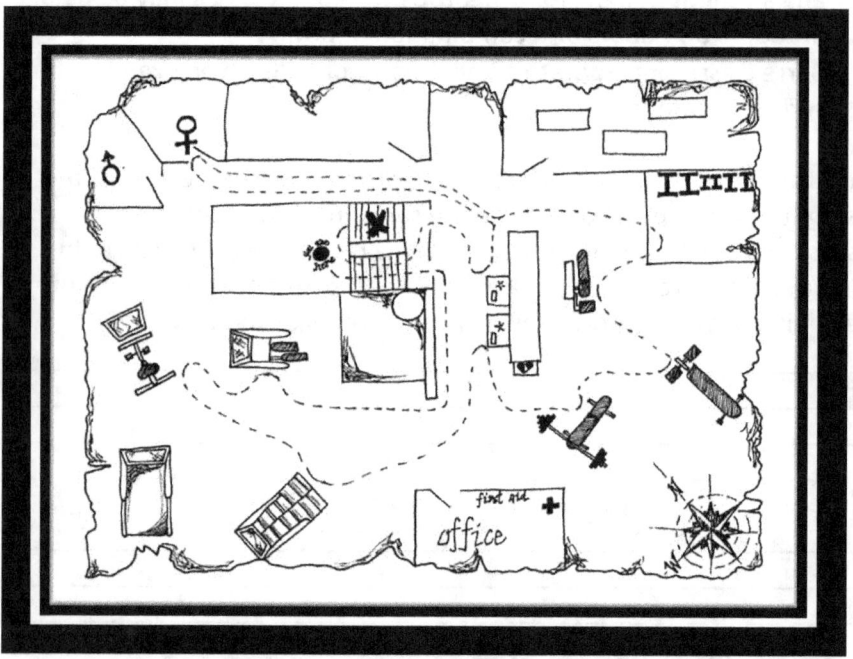

"I consider exercise to be vulgar. It makes people smell." ~Alec Quill Thornton[8]

Tip 3

Come out of the closet

It is time to come out of the closet...in clothing terms, of course.

Clothes

Exercise clothes shouldn't be too tight or too baggy.

Jocks, if your workout shorts are tight enough to show the outline of your jock strap, and uh, your package, THEY ARE TOO TIGHT. Guys and gals, make sure you cover your undergarments appropriately. Women who wear only a sports bra with their workout pants are probably breaking the rules. I've seen women escorted out of a gym because they were not properly covered. Most gyms won't allow men or women to take off their shirts indoors, no matter how warm it gets. Check the rules.

If you go the other extreme and wear baggy clothes to hide your body, just be aware that it can get caught on equipment, doorknobs, etc. Oversized clothes or layers of clothing can also cause you to overheat. A loose t-shirt can fly up with certain moves, which could be embarrassing. Your pants could get stuck on a bike pedal. It has happened. If baggy clothes are all you feel comfortable wearing at the beginning, try to re-channel your thinking. It's your call to make.

---

[8] The August Chronicle, *Slimming down can start with cleaning up*, Jan. 7, 2005

One day, you will be proud of YOU and be able to wear more formfitting exercise clothes, which allows you to see if you are using proper form. There is a difference in formfitting and tight or provocative. Dictionary.com defines provocative as "tending or serving to provoke; inciting, stimulating, irritating or vexing." It defines formfitting as "designed to fit snugly around a given shape; closefitting."

Also, make sure your pants don't droop as you exercise. Over time the elastic can wear out in a waistband. I've had to move from equipment to get out of eyesight of a butt crack or two. #gymfail9

Don't wear jeans or khakis. They are too bulky and won't move with you. <u>Wear exercise clothes</u>. There are all types. Find a style that works for you and your body.

Make-up and jewelry

Wearing make-up suitable for a night at a dance club isn't what you want to wear to the gym. The first reason is that you won't look like you are there for exercise, more like you are looking for a pickup. The other reason is that it's bad for your skin. Add a little sweat and a break-out is in your near future. If you wear mascara and eye liner, you might find it dripping down your face. Since you're working toward a healthy body, why not keep your skin healthy at the same time? Once your circulation improves, your complexion color most likely will too. Save the make-up for the night club.

The same goes for jewelry. Necklaces can get tangled; rings can make your fingers swell; bracelets can get caught on equipment. Save the bling for outside the gym. You can wear it with your soon-to-be or already smoking hot body.

Exercise accessories

Wearing a weight belt and gloves while walking around the gym might make you look strong. But, actually lifting weights is the key to looking and being strong.

If you are lifting heavy weights, a weight belt might be necessary for back support. Gloves can prevent blisters and help with gripping.

Scarves are not appropriate exercise accessories and can be hazardous. A scarf worn around your neck can get caught on equipment, so it's best to hang up the scarves before working out or leave them in your closet.

Footwear

DO NOT wear high heels to exercise. Not only will you look absurd, you might injure yourself. It really doesn't seem safe to me. I have witnessed women on cardio equipment, like the elliptical and treadmills, wearing shoes with high heels. One woman did jumping jacks in heels in between reps on resistance machines. I don't know how she didn't turn an ankle.

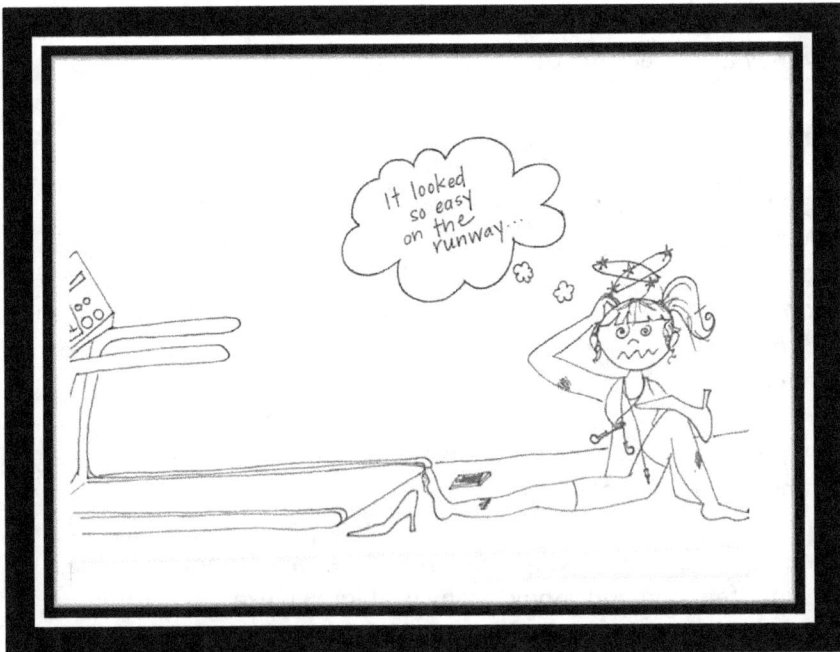

Get to the shoe store and be properly fitted with appropriate, most-likely, cross training shoes. Make sure they are comfortable and designed for your body type as well as the type of exercise you do/plan to do...and, most importantly, not high-heeled. Some sporting goods stores recommend going up a half size in exercise shoes to give some wiggle room. Shoes can wear out quickly, oftentimes within a few months, depending on how often you exercise. Consider buying two at a time. Continually check the tread and condition of your shoes to prevent injury. I used to get plantar fasciitis when my shoes got worn out. A bout or two of that and I learned quickly to replace my shoes when they needed it.

Socks are important too. Make sure they are the right thickness to suit your taste and that the heel comes up high enough to prevent blisters. The sock industry is exploding in the fitness world, so find your right fit...literally. My current favorite is Feetures!® running socks.

If you're a yogi or Pilates enthusiast, barefoot works. No one likes to see funky toes, so keep your pedicure in check. You can try to keep your socks on, but that might lead you to slip and slide in some of your poses. Some yoga studios consider the workout rooms as sacred territory and prefer that shoes not be worn in those areas. Be aware of shoe racks before entering the yoga workout room and leave shoes there. I learned this the hard way, but luckily they didn't kick me out!

Deodorant

Don't forget deodorant. If you smell bad before you begin your exercise, you'll reek by the end. Refresh your deodorant just beforehand and you'll keep people from running away. I use deodorant instead of antiperspirant so that it doesn't hinder the sweating, but keeps the odor away. Many times I have had to switch machines because the person beside me smelled so bad. #gymfail12

Go easy on perfume or cologne before working out. Sweating can intensify the scent and overwhelm others.

Overactive sweat glands necessitate wearing the type of fabric that dries quickly on your feet and your body. Many well-known exercise clothing brands have wicking fabric that pulls moisture away from your skin. Choose clothes that are comfortable, appropriate and make you feel good about yourself. You'll gain confidence the more you exercise and you'll look better too. With confidence, you won't compare yourself to the others at the gym or any place else.

Fun Fact: If you don't shower or bathe, using deodorant isn't going to cover up that smell.

More on sweat...

"Sweat cleanses from the inside. It comes from places a shower will never reach." ~ Dr. George Sheehan[9]

Tip 4

Sweat control and hydrate patrol

Sweat happens. We all do it at varying degrees.

An interesting article published in the *HuffPost Healthy Living* (August 6, 2013, Six Things You Didn't Know About Sweat) said that each of us has two to four million sweat glands. Although women have more sweat glands than men, the sweat glands in men produce more sweat. The article also said that an athlete who exercises intensely in the heat can sweat off 2 - 6% of their bodyweight.[10]

Although we might not sweat that much, we all do sweat. In *All about Sweat*,[11] Craig Freudenrich, Ph.D., wrote, "When sweat evaporates from the skin, it removes excess heat and cools you...When the water in the sweat evaporates, it leaves the salts (sodium, chloride and potassium) behind on your skin, which is why your skin tastes salty. The loss of excessive amounts of salt and water from your body can quickly dehydrate you."

---

[9] www.fuelrunning.com/running-quotes/571

[10] HUFFPOST HEALTHY LIVING, *Six Things You Didn't Know About Sweat*, Aug. 6, 2013, www.huffingtonost.com/2013/8/6/facts-about-sweat_n_3709248

[11] Freudenrich, Ph.D., Craig. *All About Sweat*, Sept. 13, 2010. HowStuffWorks.com. http://health.howstuffworks.com/skin-care/information/anatomy/how-sweat-works.htm 01 February 2015.

So, sweating is important. We can't stop it but we need to keep it to ourselves and under control. It is impolite to sling your sweat on others. It is also disgusting. You would think this would be obvious, but it isn't in many

cases. On two different occasions, I've had others sling sweat on me. One time, a girl with very long hair (not in a ponytail) was running so hard on a treadmill that she kept twisting her head and, eventually her sweat went flying through the air landing on my forearm. Another time, a man on a stair climber sweated so profusely that it dripped down to the machine where I was working out. Needless to say on both counts, I got off the equipment and went to the bathroom to wash the strangers' sweat off of me.

- Long hair should be tied back somehow. This is not a beauty contest, so you don't need to have coiffed hair at the gym.
- Wear a headband, do-rag or ball cap if needed.
- If you sweat so much while working out that it drips onto others or flies through the air at them, use a towel pppllleeaasse.
- Light gray clothing shows sweat. It practically frames it.

Of course, your goal is to sweat out the toxins and impurities while cooling off your body from rigorous exercise. Just keep the sweat on you and not others. And hit the shower ASAP!

Just as sweating is important in the body's cooling system, properly hydrating is crucial. What goes out must come back in. The more you sweat the more you need to hydrate. Drink your water before you are thirsty. Your body is made up of about 60% water. As you exercise and sweat, you'll lose some of that and you need it for energy and hydration.

Muscles hold water and hopefully you're building muscle. Many times when people think they are hungry, they are actually thirsty. So, take your water bottle and refill as necessary. Sipping at the water fountain will not be enough.

I patrol my own intake. My daily goal, based on my body and activity level, is to consume 10 – 12 glasses of water (8 ounces each).* That would take far too many trips to the water fountain, so I keep a huge water bottle with me at all times.

*Check with your doctor to get your water intake recommendations.

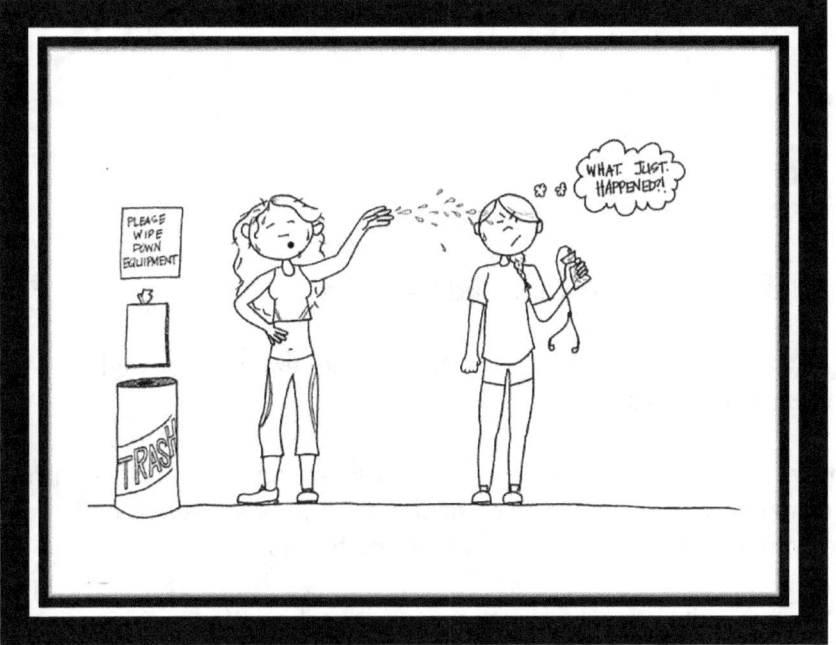

Kim Becknell Williams

Tip 5

Texting and tweeting

Texting or tweeting (we'll call it TT for short) while seated on a weight bench does not count as exercise.

Your fingers probably don't need a workout. Move your butt off the bench and let someone who is really exercising use it. Better yet, leave the phone at home or in the car so you can really focus on fitness.

Don't TT on the mats. That does not count as stretching. You're taking up valuable space and not using it appropriately.

Don't TT on the machines. You might notice that some machines indicate rules about this.

Don't TT in a class. Your instructor will probably call you out on this anyway.

So, just don't TT at the gym. You'll look like a novice. Unless you use your phone to listen to music, leave it at home. Focus, focus on exercise and fitness. While working your body, you can rest your mind.

If you have to TT while you're at the gym, go to the bathroom.

Can't resist a gym selfie on Instagram? Well, go ahead and take it quickly. You should be proud of yourself for exercising at the gym. Maybe your selfie posted on social media will inspire others...and it holds you accountable.

#TTb4youexercise

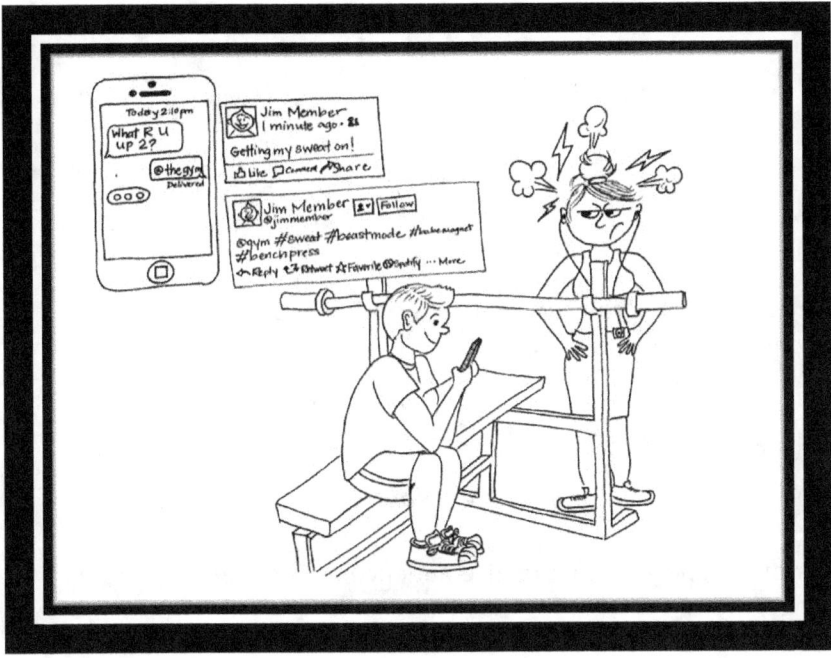

Fun Fact: Did you know that it's possible to go to the gym without posting a status about it to Facebook?

"The only reason I would take up jogging is so that I could hear heavy breathing again." ~Erma Bombeck[12]

Tip 6

P to the 4th Power

Prepare, prioritize, persist and practice patience or P Power for short, in your routine.

P1

Prepare for your workout ahead of time. Have clothes laid out, water bottle ready and iPhone/iPod ready (battery charged) to go if you listen to music while exercising. If you have children to take with you, make sure their items are packed for child care.

By packing up ahead of time, you won't run the risk of being deterred by having to pack at the last minute and you're less likely to forget something. Establish a routine and stick to it.

Have a plan for what you want your workout to be or what classes you want to take. But, be ready for a change in plans. For example, if you plan on swimming for your nightly exercise, but find that the pool is closed, revamp and choose something else (hopefully you packed more than a bathing suit). Or if your favorite cardio machine is broken, move on to something else.

---

[12] www.Quotegarden.com/running

Gym Etiquette 101

Always have a back-up plan, 'cause you never want to give up or get stuck in a rut.

Begin hydrating ahead of time.

Be prepared for unexpected sounds. If you wear headphones, especially the big ones that look like you're searching for metal in the sand, a lot of sounds will be muted. So, if you notice people looking at you, you may want to check and see if you've been singing aloud to the music.

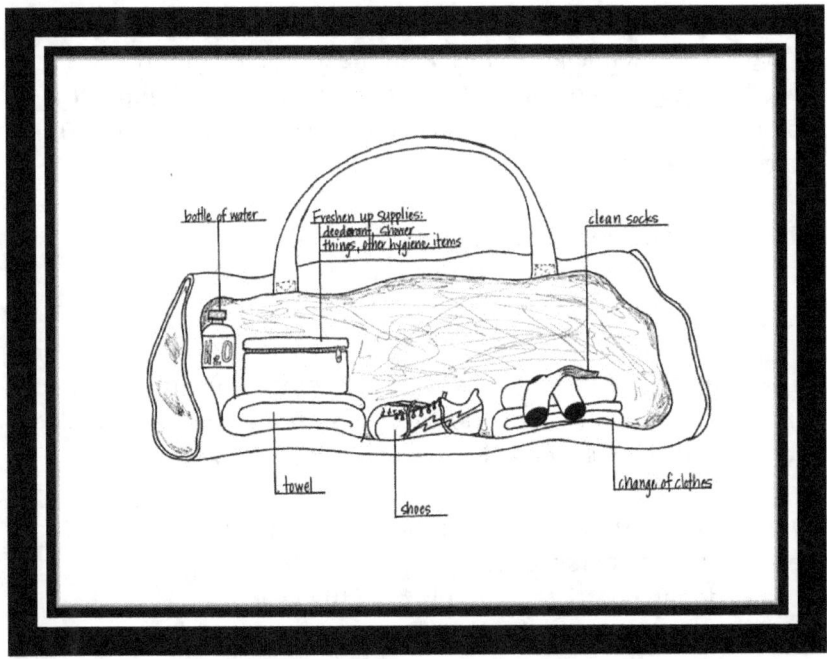

Or, you might have passed gas, farted, pooted, tooted, whatever you want to call it. Exercise, especially exercises like squats, can push that extra air or gas right out of your stomach. Try not to be horrified, it definitely happens. You can always pretend that it was someone else who did it, not you.

Are you gasping for air during your workouts? Gasping for air could be a sign that you are out of shape or are pushing yourself too hard. Gasping for air could also be a result of smoking. If you smoke, consider quitting. But, very importantly, don't grab a cigarette on your way into the gym or on the way out. If it's that necessary, wait until you're out of the gym parking lot. Most are tobacco free zones anyway. Make your lungs one of those zones as soon as you can.

P2

Prioritize what is important to your workout routine. It has to come first, not last. My husband, John, told me a story that happened at his work. The boss, at that time, put 10 free gym passes next to two dozen donuts in the employee break room. Guess what happened? All 24 donuts were taken, presumably consumed. No gym passes were used.

The house might need cleaning, clothes might need ironing or groceries might need to be bought. There's any list of excuses. If your schedule truly is busy and some things have to be done, shorten your workout. Ten or 20 minutes is more beneficial than no minutes.

Grab the gym pass first. The donut can wait.

P3

Persistence is key in the beginning because it will set the tone for the future. By continuing to strengthen your overall fitness, a routine will fall into place. It seems a lot harder to get in shape than to get out of shape.

You may come to recognize the gym rats that are regularly at the gym. They have learned the value in persistence.
I have interviewed many persistent people over the years.

- Mr. C, the 83-year old man who exercises most days of the week for an hour. He built strength after heart surgery when he began exercising at the age of 68.
- Mr. G, the 70-year old man who set the world record in his age group for powerlifting.
- Mr. Y, the 71-year old who recovered from heart surgery, then fought esophageal cancer who exercises three times a week at the gym.
- Mrs. B, the marathon runner, at the age of 52, who quit smoking and started running and lifting weights. She is well on her way to running a marathon in every state in the U.S.

- Mr. N, the 81-year old runner who started out running one mile a day five times a week for five years, eventually building up to running marathons.
- Mr. T, the blind hiker who lost his eyesight at the age of 36. He and his guide dog have hiked the Appalachian Trail, the Tahoe Rim and many other challenging trails.
- Another Mr. T, who rehabilitated himself after four motorcycle accidents with the power of yoga.

Persistence will lead to progress, but patience is key.

P4

Persistence is key in the beginning because it will set the tone for the future. By continuing to strengthen your overall fitness, a routine will fall into place. It seems a lot harder to get in shape than to get out of shape.

Patience with others will come into play when someone is committing a gymfail that bugs you. Getting angry or frustrated isn't going to do you or anybody else any good. Think positive thoughts and not about the dumbass bothering you. Hey, here's an idea...maybe you should buy that person a copy of this book, so they'll learn about gymfails!

*"Come on," said the hare, "you shall soon see what my feet are made of." ~
Aesop's Fable of the Tortoise and the Hare[13]*

Tip 7
Progress report

Whether you are making slow progress like Aesop's tortoise or fast progress like the hare, no doubt you are making progress.

Pay attention to the small, subtle signs of improvement. They are there and they will increase. If you expect big signs of improvement in a short period of time, it can be discouraging. But, much like the tortoise, slow progress is oftentimes more long-lasting than quick progress. Just like the tortoise and the hare, being quick isn't necessarily the best result.

Setting unreachable goals is one reason people give up. By setting short term attainable goals, you are more likely to hang in there. More challenging, long term goals are good to have too as long as you have short term goals.

If you were one who was intimidated by the fit bodies at the gym, hopefully you aren't thinking like that anymore. Gradually, you are likely to become one of those fit bodies, if you aren't one already.

Pat yourself on the back after a good workout. Leaving the gym after a challenging workout can create an exhilarating feeling.

---

[13] Aesopsfables.org/F134_The-Tortoise_and-the-Hare.html

If you graded yourself on progress thus far, how would you rate yourself: A - excellent, B - good, C – average, D – below average, F – failing? _____The only way to fail, is if you don't exercise at all.

To keep progressing, set up goals and a reward system. One of my motivations is competition with others, but mostly myself. Setting reasonable goals and subsequent rewards once they are reached (preferably healthy rewards) can be motivating. I have walked over to the dark side by rewarding myself with coconut ice cream stuffed in a huge waffle cone, but I try not to make it a habit.

Use this chart to set seven goals and rewards. Writing them down can make them more attainable by holding yourself accountable. More copies of the chart are included in the book's addendum.

Goal	Reward

While striving to meet your goals, you're likely to have sore muscles. Lots of topical treatments are available to help, as well as heating pads and a warm bubble bath. Try to talk your significant other or a really good friend into giving you a massage; or hire it done by a professional massage therapist. Massage has helped me keep moving, but it can be expensive.

Try foam rollers to work out the aches and pains. They can do wonders. Most gyms provide them with the stretching equipment.

Rest as needed. With all of your exercise, you should be sleeping well at night. If you find yourself excessively tired, you are overdoing it. Back off of the intensity and frequency until you feel better.

Fun Fact: A wooden rolling pin from the kitchen can roll out a lot of soreness in muscles. It's simple, cheap and it works!

If you have an injury or think you do, see a doctor.

You might be hearing some fitness terminology by now. Here are a few terms to know:

- Intervals – workouts that fluctuate between high intensity and low-level recovery mode
- HIIT – high intensity interval training
- Reps and sets – Reps are the number of repetitions in a set; so if you do 12 dumbbell curls (reps) and rest, then do 12 more, you've done 2 sets of 12 reps
- Plank (not the pirate ship kind) – an exercise where you rest on forearms and toes (or on hands with straight arms) with straight back and legs
- Core (not the apple kind) – the middle part of your body – abdominal, pelvis and back
- Circuit (not the electrical kind) – short exercises that rotate in a sequence and sometimes repeat

Beginners oftentimes gravitate to the treadmills; it's what's familiar. While you are on one, look around and watch how people use other cardio equipment. Next time, you'll be ready to try something new. You may see or be involved in some mishaps that you'll read about in the next few pages.

Most cardio equipment will include variables, like speed and incline preferences. Practice with it and see what works best for you. Some have preset programs that adjust the speed and incline for you.

Document your progress on the cardio equipment as you move forward. Be sure to alternate the days so you don't do the same exercise every day. Factor in a few days off to let your body heal too. Here's a 14-day chart to keep track of what you're doing and how you felt afterward. The same works for strength training equipment. A chart for that follows the cardio chart.

Gym Etiquette 101

See the addendum at the end of the book for additional copies of the charts.

Day	Equipment	Speed	Incline	Duration	How I Felt
1.					
2.					
3.					
4.					
5.					
6.					
7.					
8.					
9.					
10.					
11.					
12.					
13.					
14.					

Day	Equipment	Weight	Reps	Sets	How I Felt
1.					
2.					
3.					
4.					
5.					
6.					
7.					
8.					
9.					
10.					
11.					
12.					
13.					
14.					

Once your chart(s) is complete, circle the most successful days. This will give you a tracking method for the future. Do you see a pattern? Is your workout better after a day of rest or on a certain day of the week? Do you prefer certain equipment over others?

A point to consider now that you are trying new equipment:
It is rude to stand and stare at someone while waiting to use the equipment they are using. #gymfail5

Find something else to do and you'll have your turn eventually. This is very common during the holidays when people are on vacation. Many are unaccustomed to the equipment and gravitate to the one they know. Rather than try something else, they stand and wait. This is where it comes in handy to know where the free weights are to pass the time until your favorite machine is available. Or, better yet, try one of the new machines. Vary your routine. You'll see better results with variety. Trust me on that one. I speak from experience.

If you don't know how to use the equipment, ask for help. I have witnessed people falling off the arc trainer, treadmill, Jacobs ladder™ and balance ball. It never hurts to ask and it could hurt if you don't. And if you do make a mistake or fall off equipment, just get back on and laugh at yourself.

Safety comes first. But, everyone has had a little mishap; it's what makes us human. Here are a few examples that I have witnessed firsthand:

1. A gym rat was running so hard on the treadmill that she ran completely off! You may have seen videos circulating social media of the many people who fall off treadmills. That's why they have cords for a quick stop and handles for gripping.
2. Another gym rat (actually me) rolled off of a balance ball when it slipped off of a mat. I kept rolling across the gym floor along with the ball colliding with other people. A good laugh was had by all.
3. A man accidentally stepped off of the elliptical while trying to keep his iPhone from falling off the equipment while the headphones were still connected to him. He was juggling all kinds of cords! His face turned every shade of red but he never dropped his phone.
4. A woman slipped over a tree root while running trails near the gym and fell to the ground unhurt. A man running behind her started laughing. Guess what? He fell and tripped too. Karma can be a biotch.

Gym Etiquette 101

On another falling, yet inspiring, note:

I watched a hurdle event during a track meet one afternoon and witnessed ultimate determination in spite of failure. A runner started out in the lead and got his timing out of balance by the first hurdle. He knocked it over and fell on the track scraping his legs. He got up and continued running to the next hurdle only to have the same thing happen again. He knocked every hurdle down in the ¼ mile race and he fell every single time. He never gave up, crossing the finish line in last place with blood dripping down his arms and legs. An ambulance carried him away to the hospital. I have thought about that runner many times. He never quit. He didn't get embarrassed by falling over and over again. And he finished his race.

"An ounce of prevention is worth a pound of cure." ~ Benjamin Franklin[14]

Tip 8

Gym style space invaders

There are many ways to invade someone's space at the gym or to have yours invaded. You'll come to recognize some of these space invaders and may have to learn to dodge them. Just make sure you don't become one.

Conversations

Someone reading a book or wearing headphones and exercising with great intensity most likely doesn't want to hear about someone's day or the history of the pilgrims on the Mayflower. #gymfail8

If they and/or you are lifting heavy weight, they and/or you probably should be focusing on the weightlifting and not on conversation.

Judge your conversation and those with whom you converse by their mannerisms. Hopefully, they will do the same for you. Some fitness nuts engage in light conversation and some prefer to just exercise. It never hurts to communicate briefly, encouraging or asking fitness tips, but save long conversations for the water cooler. That is, unless you know someone wants to pass the time by talking to you and vice versa during the exercise routine.

Having a conversation on your phone while you are working out is equally annoying. Your jaw doesn't need exercise. #gymfail4

Gym Etiquette 101

Unless you're listening to music, put the phone away and exercise!

Paraphernalia

Many people carry a gym bag, towel or other type of accessory throughout the gym. If you take paraphernalia into an exercise room rather than lock it in a locker, be sure to keep it with you. A common complaint in weight rooms is that people will leave a gym bag on a weight machine after they have moved on to other equipment. Or they might leave a water bottle on a machine as if to reserve the equipment for later use. The gym is public and others want to exercise. Some gyms have rules against keeping bags or pocketbooks in the workout areas, due to safety issues.

No one should take up space unless they are actually using the equipment. Hogging equipment makes the pet peeve list. #gymfail10

Spitting

Spitting is inappropriate on the basketball court or in the weight room. Yes, it happens. It might help the traction on your shoes, but it doesn't help those who might trip and fall because of it in a boot camp class that follows the game.

Which leads us to...

Germs

Germs are out there and they are definitely in a gym. It's better to be safe than sorry, so always wipe down mats and equipment before and after exercise. Remember the stats earlier in the book? Not wiping down equipment is the biggest complaint of gym rats. #gymfail1

Lots of bacteria and germs thrive in the warm, humid gym conditions. This deters some germaphobes from going to the gym. #gymfail14

Exercise builds a strong immune system, but there's no point in pushing your luck.

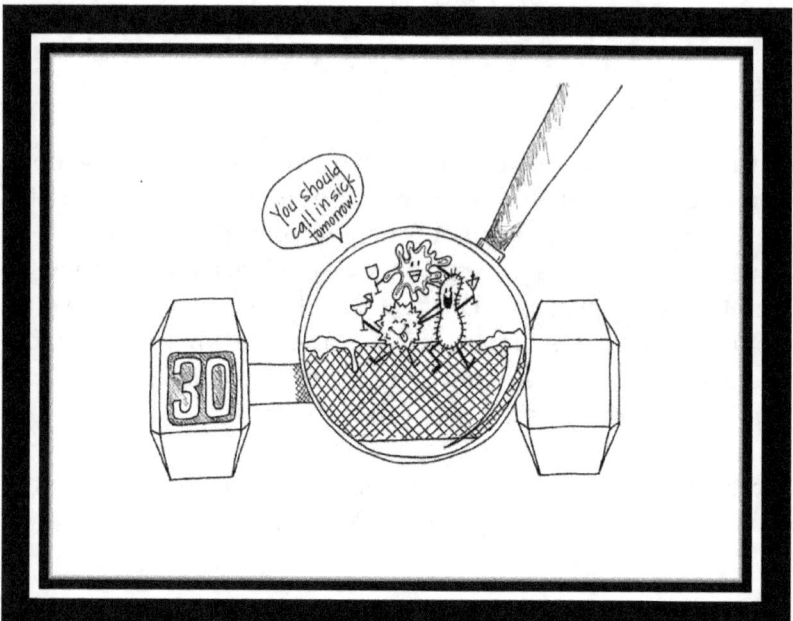

- Use an antibacterial spray and disposable paper towels or wet wipes to wipe down equipment before and after use. These are usually provided at the gym. Your sweaty gym towel doesn't count.
- If you have a cut, be sure to cover it before you exercise.
- If you are sick, stay home until you are well.
- If you choose to shower in the locker room, remember to always wear flip flops or shower shoes.
- Avoid touching your face while you're exercising.
- Wash your hands often – just like Mom taught you.
- Use the anti-bacterial soap dispensers, to clean hands in between equipment. Most gyms provide these dispensers throughout the gym and oftentimes near exit doors.

Inappropriate behavior

Basically, be considerate of others...just like in the real world. Being considerate includes never patting someone on the ass, because it makes you look like one. It is NEVER appropriate to pat someone on the ass (well, not at the gym) ...no matter how inviting their ass may be or how engaging their exercise routine might be. I had this happen to me, so I know it happens and it infuriated me.

Trying to pick up someone at the gym is frowned upon. It's a gym, not a club. #gymfail13.

Stalking someone at the gym, just like anywhere else, is not allowed.

With all the fit bodies walking around, it's hard not to notice. Consider it like eye candy - another gym benefit. No touching or stalking though. Which leads us to strutting...

"If it doesn't sweat, jiggle or pant, it's not alive." ~ Phyllis Reynolds, *The Grooming of Alice*[15]

Tip 9

Strutting your stuff

Strutting, grunting and slamming down weights are a few ways that some gym rats use to get noticed. Fitness is about exercise and conditioning, and hopefully feeling good about yourself. It's not about showing off. #gymfail11

We all have different body types and need to find a comfortable level of satisfaction in our own skin. Of course, we all want to make the most of what we have through our exercise regime. However, unlike Snow White's "mirror, mirror on the wall," it's not about "who is the fairest of them all." The mirror is there for proper form, not to stare at yourself. Everyone will see if you are primping anyway.

Stretching is important for flexibility and it is believed to help reduce the likelihood of injury. Stretching provocatively in front of the mirror while you're wearing little clothing is not appropriate in public. Cover the important parts and incorporate stretching into your workout routine.

If you must stretch in your skivvies, do it in the privacy of your own home. Study stretching techniques. Yoga bands and the wall are great ways to help you hold a stretch. It seems that when I hold a stretch for 10 seconds my brain sends a release message to my muscles to allow me to stretch a little further and longer. Warm muscles at the end of a workout will benefit from

---

[15] www.goodreads.com/quotes/1186944

some stretching. It might even help your posture, which will come in handy when you're ready to strut!

Do your work; reap the rewards; then maybe you are ready to strut a little. There is a difference between confidence and cocky.

But, please don't strut naked in the sauna or locker rooms. Wear a towel! And be sure to not leave your wet towel for others to have to move. #gymfail6

Enjoy your exercise time. Have fun with it.

And if you strut, you don't have to grunt.

If you have to grunt to impress people with how hard you are working out, you might want to reconsider the type of exercise and/or the amount of weight you are lifting. Strength training and cardio workouts need to cause a decent sweat and an occasional grunt might be heard. Continuous loud grunting might be a sign that you are exceeding your limitations or just showing off. #gymfail2

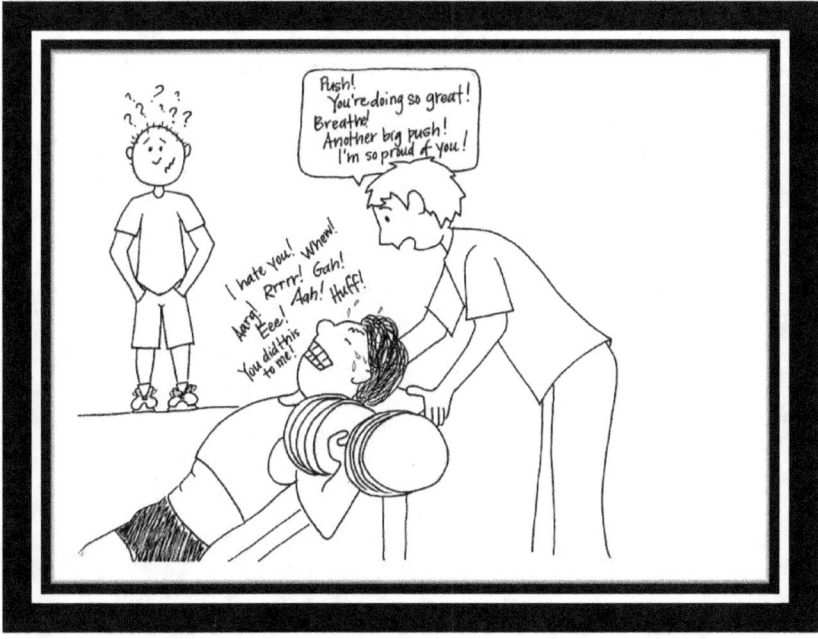

Kim Becknell Williams

Just like grunting, slamming the weights down to get noticed irritates the others in the gym. It could also land on someone's foot. #gymfail15

"Take care of your body. It's the only place you have to live." ~ Jim Rohn[16]

Tip 10

Ready, set, om!

You are ready to go. You know the basics to navigating the gym and will continue to gain confidence with experience.

Listen to your body as you progress. If you listen carefully, it will let you know what to do and what not to do, as well as what it needs. You only have one body and there are no extended warranties, so take care of it.

Find a mantra(s) suited to you, your "om" that can keep you focused. Dictionary.com defines a mantra as "a word or formula chanted or sung as an incantation or prayer." It defines om as "a mantric word thought consisting of the same three sounds representing waking, dreams and deep sleep, along with the following silence, which is fulfillment." Om is an expression used in yoga.

Repeat the mantra word or saying to yourself over and over until it sticks. I have several. One of them is very simple. When I'm challenging myself, especially in a difficult balance exercise, I say to myself, "you can do it, you can do it," over and over again throughout the exercise while I focus on one spot. Somehow the words from my mouth and the meditation in my mind convince my body that I can do it.

---

[16] Rishikajain.com/2011/05/31

Kim Becknell Williams

What will your mantra(s) be?

_____

_____

_____

_____

_____

_____

I made up a word several years ago, assitude that I use to encourage myself or someone else who is approaching competition. If you get your assitude on, you're ready to take on the opponent with focus and attitude. The opponent isn't always a person, sometimes it's a hurdle like running a marathon, competing in a mud run or simply doing one more push-up or adding five pounds to the weight bar.

Moving forward, what are your future gym goals?:

_____

_____

_____

_____

_____

_____

You are approaching the finish line.

"And will you succeed? Yes! You will, indeed! (98 and ¾ percent guaranteed)" ~ Dr. Seuss[17]

The finish line

At the end of the race, there's the finish line, the grand finale.

Crossing that finish line is always a win because you did it. Whether or not you are in first place, you have accomplished crossing the finish line at your own pace.

Years ago when my daughter ran track, the coach allowed a student with special needs to run the 800-meter event at one of the high school meets. This particular student asked if the team would buy him something from the concession stand if he won and one of the teammates nodded.

The race began and the student started running. Very quickly, he fell far behind. He fell so far back that the other runners finished the race when he still had to go all the way around the track one more time. By himself, very slowly, he ran that remaining quarter mile. When he crossed the finish line, his arms were in the air as he shouted, "I won! I won!"

And so it is with you and all of us. By keeping with your exercise program and achieving goals, you will cross a finish line many times. There may not be any fans in the stands. There may not be any medals or ribbons, but it will happen again and again. Hold your arms up and shout, "I won! I won!"

---

[17] "Oh the Places You'll Go!" by Dr. Seuss, published by Random House

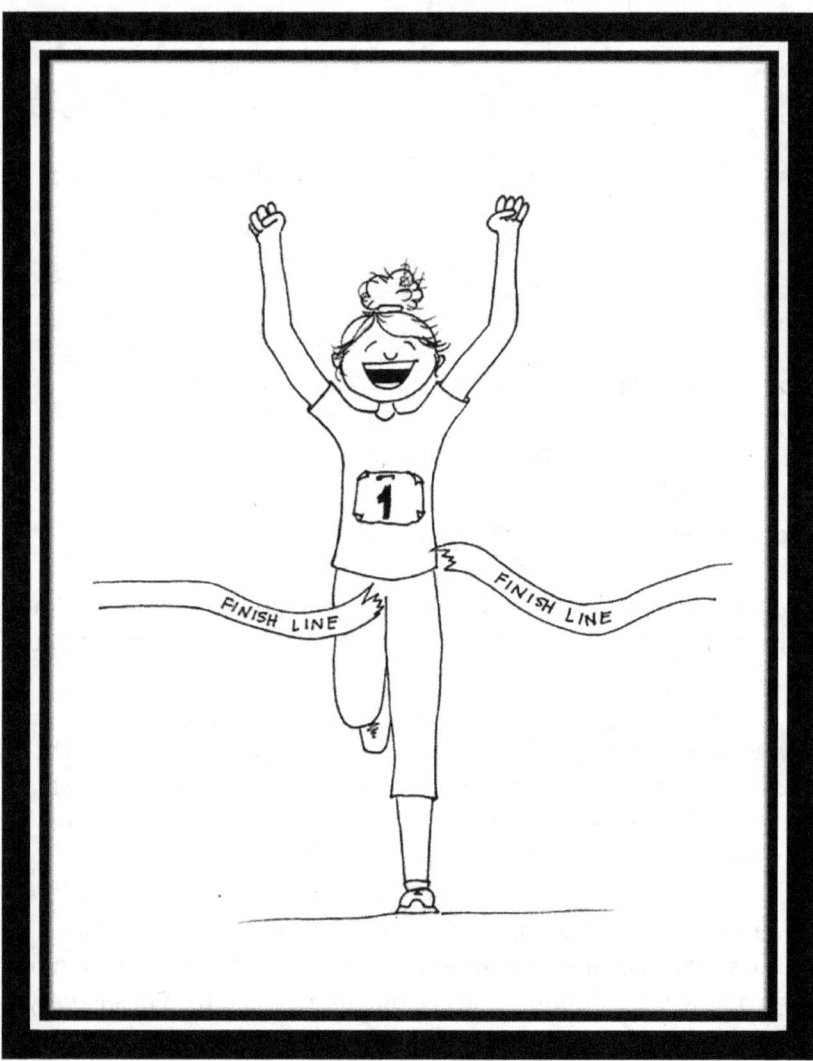

Addendum

Gym name _____Score_____

Category	Rating	Comments
Location		
Hours		
Variety of programs, classes		
Child care		
Atmosphere		
Helpful staff, instructors		
My comfort level while there		

Gym name _____Score_____

Category	Rating	Comments
Location		
Hours		
Variety of programs, classes		
Child care		
Atmosphere		
Helpful staff, instructors		
My comfort level while there		

Kim Becknell Williams

Day	Equipment	Speed	Incline	Duration	How I Felt
1.					
2.					
3.					
4.					
5.					
6.					
7.					
8.					
9.					
10.					
11.					
12.					
13.					
14.					

Day	Equipment	Weight	Reps	Sets	How I Felt
1.					
2.					
3.					
4.					
5.					
6.					
7.					
8.					
9.					
10.					
11.					
12.					
13.					
14.					

Goal	✸ Reward ✸

Goal	✸ Reward ✸

About the author

Kim Becknell Williams is a professional marketing writer and newspaper journalist, who has written for numerous newspapers and magazines.

She is also a certified master level personal trainer with specialties in resistance training, sport nutrition and endurance training through National Federation of Professional Trainers (NFPT).

And, she is addicted to her gym workouts. Combining her love of writing and exercise, she wrote this book to encourage others toward living a fitness lifestyle and to feel comfortable in a gym.

Follow her on social media and the web:

On Facebook: Kim Becknell Williams – Freelance Writer
Twitter: @kimbecknellwil4